Mediterranean Diet Cookbook

Easy and Delicious Mediterranean Diet
Recipes for Weight Loss and Better Health

Melinda Nelson

Paperback ISBN: 978-1-951548-73-5

Table of Contents

CHAPTER ONE...1

Introduction to the Mediterranean Diet.......................................1

Principles of the Mediterranean Diet...1
Health Benefits 3
Foods to Enjoy on the Mediterranean Diet...................................3
Foods to Avoid on the Mediterranean Diet 5

CHAPTER TWO..6

Breakfast 6

Oats with Banana and Strawberry 6
Multigrain Hot Cereal..7
Scrambled Eggs with Spinach 8
Baked Eggs with Feta Cheese and Olives 9
Carrot Bread 11
Walnut Muffins 12
Toast with Avocado..14
Mediterranean Couscous 15
Tapioca Pancakes 16
Whole Wheat Pancakes with Greek Yogurt.................................17
Veggie and Herb Frittata 18
Fruit and Nut Breakfast Salad 20
Simple Smoothie 21

CHAPTER THREE...23

Vegetables and Beans 23

Pasta and Artichoke Salad 23
Rice and Bean Salad 24
Fruity Wheat Berry Salad...25
Tomatoes Stuffed with Cheese and Olives...................................27

Avocado and Egg Sandwich 28

Nutty Quinoa 29

Bean and Farro Stew 30

Quinoa Casserole..31

Fully Loaded Baked Potato 33

Stuffed Zucchini 34

Phyllo Spinach Pie 36

Vegetarian Chili 37

CHAPTER FOUR 39

Poultry and Meats 39

Chicken Pasta 39

Chicken Soup with Orzo 40

Balsamic Chicken Wrap 42

Roasted Chicken...43

Baked Chicken Wings with Tzatziki Dipping Sauce 44

Balsamic Chicken and Beans 47

Turkey Sausage and Peppers 48

Slow Cooker Mediterranean Short Ribs..................49

Grilled Steak..50

Spicy Roasted Leg of Lamb 51

CHAPTER FIVE..53

Fish and Seafood..53

Spicy Shrimp Salad 53

Salmon Spinach Salad...55

Tuna Salad with Capers...56

Pasta with Shrimp..57

Lemon Pepper Cod with Chickpeas 58

Mediterranean Baked Salmon 59

Pepper Tilapia with Spinach 60

Baked Snapper with Olives 61

CHAPTER SIX..63

Snacks 63

    Grilled Figs and Goat Cheese....................................63

    Caprese Kebobs...64

    Spicy Olives...65

    Marinated Olives & Feta Cheese................................66

    Roasted Eggplant Dip...67

    Basic Hummus..68

    Feta Hummus...69

    Spiced Nuts..71

    Fruity Nut Bars...72

    Tomato Sandwiches with Basil 73

    Date Wraps 74

CHAPTER SEVEN 75

Dessert 75

    Galatopita 75

    Apples with Parmesan 76

    Pudding Parfait..77

    Fruit and Yogurt Lasagna...78

    Banana Balls..79

    Chocolate Hazelnut Baklava 80

CHAPTER EIGHT 82

Mediterranean Diet Instant Pot Recipes 82

    Good Morning Quinoa 82

    Crustless Seafood Quiche...83

    Quick Vegetable Curry...84

    Chipotle Black Beans 86

    Spiced Okra...87

    Spinach with Tomatoes 88

    Lemon Garlic Chicken 89

    Cilantro Lime Drumsticks..91

    Mediterranean Beef 92

Tasty Fish Stew 93
Coconut Curry Tilapia 96
Mediterranean Calamari 98
Orange Salmon 99
Instant Pot Hummus 100
Wine Poached Figs on Yogurt Crème 101

Final Thoughts **102**

x

CHAPTER ONE

Introduction to the Mediterranean Diet

The word "diet" comes from the Latin diaeta and the Greek diaita, and it means "way of life." With this thinking, a diet ceases to be a punishment, or a series of limitations, but a means to enjoy each day to the fullest.

People living in Mediterranean countries such as Greece, Italy, Spain, France, and Morocco tend to live healthy and long lives. One of the factors contributing to this excellent health is diet. The Mediterranean Diet is an eating plan developed from the lifestyle habits of people living in the Mediterranean countries. After studying the Mediterranean Diet, nutritionists began recommending that people with weight management issues, or anyone trying to stay lean and healthy, adopt similar eating styles.

Principles of the Mediterranean Diet

There is no mystery as to why the Mediterranean Diet is so beneficial. Compared to the average American diet, it's low in sugar, salt, unhealthy fats, and processed foods. There are several important principles of the Mediterranean Diet that you need to understand if you're going to have success with it.

First Principle: Plant-Based Foods Are Best
You're going to build your meals from fresh, seasonal fruits and vegetables, as well as legumes, nuts, and whole grains. You'll want to use herbs and spices liberally too.

Second Principle: Oil is Better than Butter

Fats are okay when you're following the Mediterranean Diet, but eating the right kinds of fats is key. That means trading in your butter, or your butter substitute, for something natural and heart-healthy, like olive oil. If you look at the label on your olive oil in your pantry or at the grocery store, you'll notice it probably comes from a Mediterranean country. It's used liberally in their diet, and you need to get into the habit of doing that too.

Third Principle: Smart Protein Choices
Although red meat is consumed on the Mediterranean Diet, it's not eaten every day. Instead, you should get your protein sources from poultry and fish. Incorporate beef and other types of red meats only once a week. Eggs and cheese also provide you with good protein options, and they are healthier than red meat.

Fourth Principle: Eat According to the Season
You won't find many people in Mediterranean countries eating foods that aren't seasonal. They choose the freshest food possible, and they know that in order to find the healthiest and best tasting options, they have to eat what is grown locally and seasonally. Each meal should include whatever is available at the time, such as squash in the fall and tomatoes in the summer.

Fifth Principle: Skip the Salt
A lot of Mediterranean food doesn't require salt because the recipes are full of natural, flavorful, and healthy herbs and spices. Substitute fresh or dried herbs and spices for salt whenever you can.

Here's a bonus principle: Red wine is a staple at every meal in Mediterranean countries. Enjoy a glass with your meal once in a while.

Health Benefits

There are a number of health benefits that come with the Mediterranean Diet. The most important benefit for most people is weight loss. You won't lose weight because you've dramatically reduced your caloric intake; instead you'll lose weight because you are eating foods that your body needs. When you're eating foods that are high in vitamins, minerals, fiber, and protein, your body will know exactly what to do with them. This keeps your metabolism high, naturally burning and flushing fat. As your body adjusts to this new way of eating, you'll shed pounds quickly and permanently. The Diet is also a good choice for people who have chronic illnesses associated with weight troubles. If your weight has been a medical issue for you, talk to your doctor about the Mediterranean plan to see if it would be a good match for your weight goals.

Your heart will also benefit greatly from this eating plan. As the Diet limits salt intake, many people have noticed that their blood pressure is lowered and their cholesterol counts are improved. Studies have shown that people who eat according to the Mediterranean Diet have a lower risk of cardiovascular events such as heart attacks and strokes. It may also reduce the risks of certain types of cancer, Parkinson's disease, and Alzheimer's.

Foods to Enjoy on the Mediterranean Diet

When you're following this eating plan, you'll be eating all of your favorite fruits and vegetables in abundance. Enjoy berries, melon, grapes, apples, and citrus fruits. Experiment with different vegetables, and eat as much eggplant, broccoli, cauliflower, spinach, kale, artichokes, green beans, olives, avocados, and tomatoes as you want. Beans are a big part of the Mediterranean diet too. Eat black beans, red beans, white beans, and lima beans.

You should also enjoy nuts and seeds. Some excellent snacks that are Mediterranean-friendly include almonds, dates, figs, sunflower seeds, and walnuts.

High fiber foods such as whole grain bread, brown rice, lentils, and wheat are also encouraged while you're eating on this plan. You should also incorporate oils such as olive oil and avocado oil. Olive oil is a great fat to cook with and you can use extra virgin olive oil to dress your salads and vegetables. Vinegars such as balsamic vinegar are also excellent and do a wonderful job of adding flavor to meats, cheeses, and veggies.

Your protein sources should consist of chicken, other poultry, fish, and eggs. Turkey, guinea fowl, shrimp, salmon, cod, and sardines are great-tasting foods that also pack a healthy punch. All of your meals will ideally include one protein source and at least one serving each of vegetables and fruits.

The following small steps can help you get started on the Mediterranean Diet:

- Eat fruits or vegetables with every meal, including snack time.
- Go for whole grain bread, whole grain pasta, and brown or wild rice instead of white rice.
- Swap hamburger night for seafood night at least two times each week.
- Choose olive oil instead of margarine or butter.
- Drink skim milk instead of whole milk, and eat non-fat yogurt instead of full fat yogurt.
- Do you need a crunchy snack? Choose carrots and celery instead of crackers and pretzels.
- Experiment with ancient grains such as bulgur and quinoa.
- Use spices and herbs to flavor food instead of fat and salt.

Foods to Avoid on the Mediterranean Diet

There is no place in this eating plan for packaged, processed foods, or anything containing unnatural ingredients such as trans fats. You'll have to skip the fast food lines and forget the microwaved meals. Sweets such as cookies, cakes, and candies should only be enjoyed in moderation, and not as everyday snacks or desserts. Limit your red meat intake to one serving per week, and avoid butter, salt, and other fats that are unhealthy.

If you want to adopt the Mediterranean eating plan, the first thing you need to learn is how to shop and cook like a Mediterranean. Get to know the fish expert and the produce suppliers at your grocery store. Visit local farmers' markets and shop for organic ingredients, or try to grow your own food. You'll find that you'll enjoy what you get to put on your plate. The 75 easy and delicious recipes in this book will help you transition to and enjoy the Mediterranean Diet.

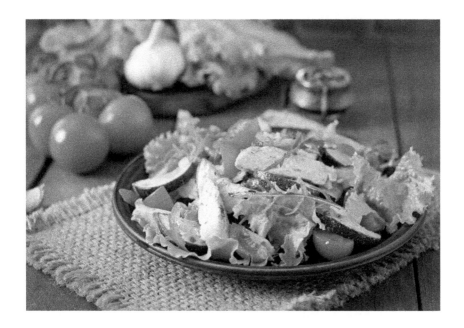

CHAPTER TWO

Breakfast

Oats with Banana and Strawberry

Eating the Mediterranean way means enjoying lots of fresh fruit. There's no cooking involved, just lots of luscious flavors.

Makes 10 servings
Ingredients:
3 cups rolled oats
¼ cup walnuts, chopped
¼ cup dates, chopped
¼ cup shredded coconut
4 tablespoons chia seeds
2 bananas, sliced
4 strawberries, sliced
3 cups almond milk
2 tablespoons maple syrup

Directions:
1. Combine all dry ingredients in a bowl.
2. Place the fruit in a food processor and pulse until they liquefy.
3. Mix the fruit into the dry ingredients.
4. Add the almond milk and maple syrup and mix everything together.
5. Cover the bowl and refrigerate overnight.
6. Enjoy breakfast in the morning. If desired, add extra fruit or nuts.

Nutritional Information (Per Serving)
Calories: 355
Fat: 23.2 g
Sat Fat: 16.4 g
Carbohydrates: 35 g
Fiber: 7.5 g
Sugar: 11.1 g
Protein: 7.3 g
Sodium: 13 mg

Multigrain Hot Cereal

Makes 8 servings

Ingredients:

½ cup pearl barley
½ cup red wheat berries
½ cup brown rice
¼ cup steel cut oats
3 tablespoons quinoa
¼ teaspoon kosher salt
1½ quarts water

Directions:

1. Add all ingredients to a saucepan, stir to mix and bring to a boil.

2. Reduce the heat to low and allow to simmer for 45 minutes giving it an occasional stir.

3. The cereal can be refrigerated and reheated for quick breakfasts or snacks throughout the week.

Nutritional Information (Per Serving)
Calories: 118
Fat: 1.0 g
Sat Fat: 0 g
Carbohydrates: 23.6 g

Fiber: 4.3 g
Sugar: 0.6 g
Protein: 4.0 g
Sodium: 74.6 mg

Scrambled Eggs with Spinach

Boring scrambled eggs? These eggs will reawaken your taste buds.

Makes 5 servings

Ingredients:

10 eggs
½ cup light cream
2 tablespoons olive oil
1 garlic clove, minced
2 cups tomatoes, diced
2 cups baby spinach (fresh, not frozen)
¼ cup parmesan cheese, shredded
Salt and pepper to taste

Directions:

1. Whisk together the eggs, cream, salt, and pepper in a bowl.
2. Heat the oil in a skillet over medium heat and sauté the garlic for 30 seconds.
3. Add the tomatoes and spinach and keep stirring until the spinach leaves are wilted.
4. Transfer to a bowl and cover with aluminum foil.
5. Cook the eggs in the same skillet. Don't stir or "scramble."
6. When the eggs are set but still soft, top with the parmesan cheese and spinach.

Nutritional Information (Per Serving)
Calories: 242
Fat: 19.3 g

Sat Fat: 6.6 g
Carbohydrates: 4.6 g
Fiber: 1.1 g
Sugar: 2.6 g
Protein: 13.9 g

Baked Eggs with Feta Cheese and Olives

This is a great way to enjoy eggs and vegetables at breakfast.

Makes 4 servings
Ingredients:
3 tablespoons olive oil
1 cup onions, chopped
2 garlic cloves, minced
8 eggs, beaten
¼ cup light cream
2 ounces feta cheese, crumbled
8 olives, pitted and sliced (preferably kalamata)
Salt and pepper to taste
½ cup seasoned croutons, crushed
3 tablespoons shredded parmesan cheese

Directions:
1. Preheat the broiler.
2. Heat 2 tablespoon of olive oil in a non-stick skillet.
3. Sauté the onion and garlic for about 5 minutes.
4. In a bowel, whip together the eggs and cream.
5. Add the feta cheese, sliced olives, salt, and pepper.
6. Pour the egg mixture on top of the onions.
7. Cook on low heat until the eggs are just about set.

8. In another bowl, mix the croutons, parmesan cheese, and 1 tablespoon olive oil.

9. Top the eggs with the cheese mix.

10. Place in the oven and broil for 2 minutes or until the top is golden.

Nutritional Information (Per Serving)
Calories: 338
Fat: 27.6 g
Sat Fat: 8.7 g
Carbohydrates: 8.5 g
Fiber: 1.2 g
Sugar: 2.7 g
Protein: 15.7 g
Sodium: 488 mg

Carrot Bread

Makes 8 servings

Ingredients:

2 cups almond flour

1 teaspoon baking powder

1 tablespoon cumin seeds

½ teaspoon salt

3 large eggs

2 tablespoons olive oil

1 tablespoon apple cider vinegar

3 cups carrots, peeled and grated

½ teaspoon fresh ginger, peeled and grated finely

¼ cup raisins

Directions:

1. Preheat the oven to 350 degrees F.

2. Line a loaf pan with parchment paper.

3. In a large bowl, add almond flour, baking powder, cumin seeds, and salt and mix well.

4. In another bowl, add the eggs, olive oil, and vinegar, and beat until well combined.

5. Add egg mixture to the flour mixture, and mix until well combined.

6. Gently fold in carrot, ginger, and raisins.

7. Place the mixture into the prepared loaf pan.

8. Bake for about 1 hour until a toothpick inserted in the center comes out clean.

Nutritional Information (Per Serving)

Calories: 253

Fat: 19.4 g

Sat Fat: 2.1 g

Carbohydrates: 14.8 g

Fiber: 4.6 g

Sugar: 6.0 g
Protein: 9.1 g
Sodium: 268 mg

Walnut Muffins

These delicious muffins can be frozen, so you can have them on hand when you're rushed in the morning. Just take one out of the freezer and pop it in the oven.

Makes 6 servings
Ingredients:
2 cups quinoa flour
2 teaspoons baking powder
2 teaspoons cinnamon
Dash of salt
4 eggs
½ cup honey
1 banana, mashed
1 apple, diced or grated
½ cup walnuts, chopped

Directions:
1. Preheat oven to 350 degrees F.
2. Insert paper liners into a 12-cup muffin pan.
3. In one bowl, mix the flour, baking powder, cinnamon, and salt.
4. In another bowl, blend the eggs, honey, and banana.
5. Fold the egg mixture into the flour and stir in the apple and walnuts.
6. Pour the batter equally into the muffin cups.
7. Bake for 30 minutes.

Nutritional Information (Per Serving)
Calories: 263
Fat: 9.8 g
Sat Fat: 1.3 g
Carbohydrates: 40.1 g
Fiber: 3.2 g
Sugar: 28.6 g
Protein: 8 g
Sodium: 74 mg

Toast with Avocado

Skip the butter and the jelly and have some toast that's really worth eating - topped with an avocado spread.

Makes 4 servings

Ingredients:

4 slices of high fiber, whole grain bread

2 small avocados, peeled with stone removed

2 ounces feta cheese, crumbled

2 tablespoons fresh lemon juice

2 tablespoons fresh mint, chopped

Pepper to taste

Directions:

1. Toast your bread in a toaster or broiler.

2. Mash the avocado with a fork until it's smooth. Add the cheese, lemon juice, and mint.

3. Spread the mixture over your toasted bread and garnish with a little black pepper and any extra mint.

Nutritional Information (Per Serving)

Calories: 353

Fat: 20.4 g

Sat Fat: 5.7 g

Carbohydrates: 37.9 g

Fiber: 12.8 g

Sugar: 8.5 g

Protein: 11.6 g

Sodium: 464 mg

Mediterranean Couscous

You'll never crave another donut once you've tasted this Mediterranean delight.

Makes 4 servings

Ingredients:

3 cups milk

1 cinnamon stick

1½ cups uncooked couscous

¼ cup dried apricots, diced

¼ cup dried grapes or cherries

4 teaspoons honey

Dash of salt

4 teaspoons olive oil

Directions:

1. Heat the milk in a pan with the cinnamon stick just below the boiling point.

2. Remove the pan from the stove and add the couscous, dried fruit, 2 teaspoons of the honey and salt.

3. Cover the pan and let sit for 15 minutes.

4. Discard the cinnamon stick.

5. Top the couscous with the remaining honey and olive oil.

Nutritional Information (Per Serving)

Calories: 415

Fat: 8.9 g

Sat Fat: 3 g

Carbohydrates: 69.7 g

Fiber: 3.6 g

Sugar: 17.6 g

Protein: 14.6 g

Sodium: 132 mg

Tapioca Pancakes

Makes 6 servings

Ingredients:

½ cup tapioca flour

½ cup almond flour

½ teaspoon red chili powder

¼ teaspoon salt

Black pepper to taste

1 cup coconut milk

½ red onion, chopped

¼ teaspoon fresh ginger, minced

1 serrano pepper, seeded and minced

½ cup fresh parsley leaves, chopped

2 tablespoons olive oil

Directions:

1. In a large bowl, mix together flours and spices. Add the coconut milk, and mix until well combined.

2. Fold in the onion, ginger, serrano pepper, and cilantro.

3. Lightly grease a large non-stick skillet with oil, and heat over medium heat.

4. Add about ¼ cup of mixture, and tilt the pan to spread it evenly in the skillet. Cook for about 3–4 minutes for both sides.

5. Repeat with the remaining mixture.

6. Serve with your desired topping.

Nutritional Information (Per Serving)
Calories: 146
Fat: 10.1 g
Sat Fat: 1.8 g
Carbohydrates: 13.1 g
Fiber: 1.4 g
Sugar: 1.4 g
Protein: 2.4 g

Sodium: 107 mg

Whole Wheat Pancakes with Greek Yogurt

Top these beauties with nuts, berries, yogurt, or syrup.

Makes 6 servings

Ingredients:
1 cup rolled oats
½ cup whole wheat flour
1 tablespoon flax seeds
1 teaspoon baking soda
Dash of salt
2 eggs
2 cups plain Greek yogurt
3 tablespoons honey
4 tablespoons vegetable oil

Directions:
1. Place the oats, flour, flax seeds, baking soda, and salt in a food processor and blend well.
2. Add the eggs, yogurt, honey, and 2 tablespoons of oil and blend until the batter is smooth.
3. Allow the batter to sit for 30 minutes.
4. Heat ½ tablespoon of oil in a non-stick skillet and add ¼ cup batter per pancake.
5. Cook for 2 minutes, flip the pancakes, and cook for another 2 minutes.
6. Repeat until all of the batter has been used.
7. Serve pancakes with topping of choice.

Nutritional Information (Per Serving)

Calories: 272
Fat: 11.9 g
Sat Fat: 2.5 g
Carbohydrates: 33.3 g
Fiber: 3 g
Sugar: 14.8 g
Protein: 9 g
Sodium: 320 mg

Veggie and Herb Frittata

It sounds like a fancy breakfast dish, but frittatas are surprisingly easy, and this one includes red peppers which are great for your immune system as well as your waistline.

Makes 2 servings

Ingredients:

5 eggs

1 red bell pepper, sliced

2 cloves of garlic, minced

3 leaves of fresh basil

1 sprig of fresh rosemary

1 tablespoon olive oil

¼ cup shredded mozzarella cheese

Salt and pepper to taste

Directions:

1. Preheat broiler.

2. In a small oven-proof pan, heat olive oil. Add bell pepper and garlic and cook for 5 minutes.

3. Whisk eggs together in a small bowl.

4. Pour the eggs on top of the peppers and garlic in the pan. Top with feta cheese and herbs, then place the pan in the oven for about 5 minutes, until the eggs set and the cheese starts to bubble.

5. Season with salt and pepper.

Nutritional Information (Per Serving)
Calories: 251
Fat: 18.8 g
Sat Fat: 4.8 g
Carbohydrates: 6.6 g
Fiber: 0.9 g
Sugar: 3.9 g
Protein: 15.7 g

Fruit and Nut Breakfast Salad

There's nothing easier to prepare for breakfast than fruit salad. You can even double or triple this recipe and keep it in the fridge for breakfast all week long or an easy go-to snack.

Makes 4 servings

Ingredients:

1 cup red grapes

1 cup green grapes

½ cup blueberries

2 cups watermelon, chopped

2 cups cantaloupe, chopped

½ cup walnuts

½ cup almonds

½ cup raisins

Directions:

1. Combine all the fruit together and toss.

2. Add the walnuts and almonds. This can be served with a side of your favorite Greek yogurt.

Nutritional Information (Per Serving)

Calories: 322

Fat: 15.6 g

Sat Fat: 1.1 g

Carbohydrates: 44.3 g

Fiber: 5.1 g

Sugar: 33.8 g

Protein: 8.5 g

Sodium: 17 mg

Simple Smoothie

If you simply cannot imagine eating a breakfast that isn't on the run, this smoothie recipe will keep you mobile as well as fed. Mix up the fruit selections if others are in season.

Makes 1 serving

Ingredients:

1 medium banana

1 cup strawberries

1 cup raspberries

½ cup plain yogurt

1 tablespoon honey

½ cup ice

Directions:

1. Mix all of the ingredients into a blender and combine on high until frothy.

Nutritional Information (Per Serving)

Calories: 366

Fat: 3.1 g

Sat Fat: 1.4 g

Carbohydrates: 78.6 g

Fiber: 14 g

Sugar: 52.8 g

Protein: 10.8 g

Sodium: 94 mg

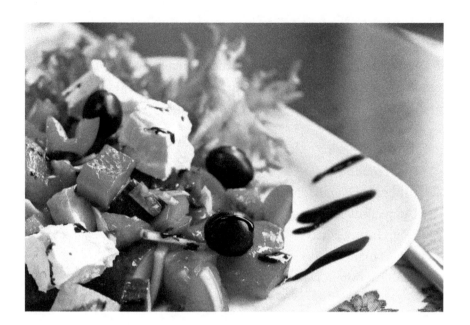

CHAPTER THREE

Vegetables and Beans

Pasta and Artichoke Salad

This salad has a zing that doesn't need any mayonnaise.

Makes 4 servings

Ingredients:

8 ounces spiral pasta

¼ cup frozen peas, thawed

1 tablespoon lemon juice

3 teaspoons olive oil

1 can chopped artichoke hearts

8 ounces mozzarella cheese, diced

⅓ cup roasted red bell pepper, chopped

Directions:

1. Cook the pasta according to directions. When done, add the peas.

2. Mix the lemon juice and olive oil together in a bowl. Stir in the remaining ingredients.

3. Mix in the pasta and peas.

4. Serve warm or at room temperature.

Nutritional Information (Per Serving)

Calories: 435

Fat: 14.5 g

Sat Fat: 6.7 g

Carbohydrates: 51.4 g

Fiber: 4 g

Sugar: 2.9 g

Protein: 25.1 g

Sodium: 442 mg

Rice and Bean Salad

Makes 6 servings

Ingredients:

1 cup rice

¾ cup sun-dried tomatoes

2 tablespoons olive oil

3 cups baby spinach

3 garlic cloves, minced

6 ounces feta cheese, crumbled

1 teaspoon oregano

Salt and pepper to taste

15 ounces garbanzo beans, drained

2 tablespoons toasted pine nuts

Directions:

1. Prepare the rice according to package directions and set aside.

2. Soak the sun-dried tomatoes in a cup of boiling water for 30 minutes, then dice.

3. Sauté the spinach and garlic in 1 tablespoon of the olive oil until the spinach is wilted.

4. In a bowl, combine the remaining ingredients (except the pine nuts), the rice, and the tomatoes.

5. Spoon the remaining tablespoon of olive oil over the salad and toss.

6. Top with the pine nuts.

Nutritional Information (Per Serving)
Calories: 515
Fat: 17.3 g
Sat Fat: 5.6 g

Carbohydrates: 71.3 g
Fiber: 13.6 g
Sugar: 9.6 g
Protein: 21.1 g

Fruity Wheat Berry Salad

Makes 4 servings

Ingredients for the Salad:

2 cups water

1 cup wheat berries

1 cup mango, peeled, pitted, and cubed

1 cup pineapple, chopped

1 red bell pepper, seeded and chopped

2 scallions, chopped

½ cup fresh mint leaves, chopped

½ cup cranberries

½ cup walnuts, toasted and chopped

Ingredients for the Dressing:

1 tablespoon fresh ginger, minced

½ cup plain 2% Greek yogurt

3 tablespoons honey

½ teaspoon balsamic vinegar

¼ teaspoon salt

Black pepper to taste

Directions:

1. In a pan, add water and wheat berries, and bring to a boil. Cover and simmer for about 35 minutes.

2. Remove from heat, and set aside to cool completely.

3. In a large bowl, add wheat berries and remaining ingredients and mix.

4. In a small bowl, add dressing ingredients, and beat well.

5. Place dressing over salad mixture, and toss to coat well.

6. Serve immediately.

Nutritional Information (Per Serving)
Calories: 379
Fat: 11.5 g
Sat Fat: 1.3 g
Carbohydrates: 66.5 g
Fiber: 10.2 g
Sugar: 26.3 g
Protein: 22.8 g
Sodium: 173 mg

Tomatoes Stuffed with Cheese and Olives

A light and healthy lunch that's meant to be savored.

Makes 2 servings

Ingredients:

2 large tomatoes

½ cup garlic croutons

1 ounce goat cheese

⅓ cup kalamata olives, pitted and chopped

1½ tablespoons Italian salad dressing

1½ tablespoons chopped basil

Directions:

1. Preheat the broiler horizontally.

2. Cut the tomatoes in half and remove the pulp and seeds.

3. Dice the pulp and transfer to a bowl. Add the remaining ingredients and mix.

4. Spoon the filling into the tomato shells.

5. Transfer to a baking sheet and broil for 5 minutes.

Nutritional Information (Per Serving)

Calories: 250

Fat: 19.6 g

Sat Fat: 5.8 g

Carbohydrates: 14.5 g

Fiber: 3.2 g

Sugar: 8.5 g

Protein: 6.5 g

Sodium: 279 mg

Avocado and Egg Sandwich

The avocado makes this a rich, luscious sandwich.

Makes 2 servings

Ingredients:

1 avocado, diced

1 tablespoon lemon juice

2 eggs, hard-boiled and chopped

3 scallions, chopped

4 tablespoon corn kernels

1 tomato, diced

1 tablespoon olive oil

Salt and pepper to taste

Directions:

1. Add the lemon juice to the avocado.

2. Stir in the remaining ingredients.

3. Serve with bread

Nutritional Information (Per Serving)

Calories: 382

Fat: 31.6 g

Sat Fat: 6.6 g

Carbohydrates: 19.1 g

Fiber: 8.5 g

Sugar: 3 g

Protein: 9.2 g

Nutty Quinoa

Makes 4 servings

Ingredients:

1 tablespoon extra-virgin olive oil

1 teaspoon curry powder

½ teaspoon ground cumin

1 cup quinoa, rinsed and drained

1 cup vegetable broth

1 cup water

¾ cup almonds, toasted

½ cup raisins

¾ cup fresh parsley, chopped

Directions:

1. In a medium pan, heat oil over medium-high heat. Add curry powder and cumin, and sauté for 1–2 minutes.

2. Add quinoa and sauté for 2 minutes.

3. Add vegetable broth and water, and stir to combine. Cover and reduce heat to low. Simmer for 20 minutes.

4. Remove from heat and set aside, covered for about 5 minutes.

5. Just before serving, add almonds and raisins, and toss to coat.

6. Drizzle with lemon juice and serve.

Nutritional Information (Per Serving)
Calories: 408
Fat: 19.8 g
Sat Fat: 1.6 g
Carbohydrates: 50.6 g
Fiber: 7.0 g
Sugar: 12.7 g
Protein: 12.4 g
Sodium: 254 mg

Bean and Farro Stew

Makes 5 servings

Ingredients:

2 tablespoon olive oil

1 onion, chopped

2 celery stalks, chopped

3 garlic cloves, minced

3 cups vegetable broth

2 cups water

2 cups tomatoes, chopped

1 cup farro

1 teaspoon oregano

1 bay leaf

A dash of salt

5 cups kale, chopped

1 can cannellini beans

1 tablespoon lemon juice

Feta cheese

Directions:

1. Use a Dutch oven to sauté the onion, celery, and garlic in the olive oil for 4 minutes.

2. Pour in the vegetable broth, water, tomatoes, farro, and seasoning (not the lemon juice). Let it come to a boil.

3. Immediately lower the heat and simmer, covered for 20 minutes.

4. Add the kale, then cook for another 10 minutes.

5. Stir in the cannellini beans and cook for 5 minutes.

6. Discard the bay leaf and add the lemon juice. Mix and serve.

Nutritional Information (Per Serving)
Calories: 286
Fat: 7 g

Sat Fat: 1.1 g
Carbohydrates: 42.1 g
Fiber: 12.4 g
Sugar: 4.2 g
Protein: 16.1 g
Sodium: 544 mg

Quinoa Casserole

Enjoy healthy quinoa and lentils in this casserole.

Makes 8 servings

Ingredients:

2½ cups quinoa, cooked according to package instructions
2 cups lentils, cooked according to package instructions
1 onion, diced
3 garlic cloves, minced
1 tablespoon olive oil
10 ounces fresh spinach
2 cups tomatoes, diced
2 eggs
½ cup plain Greek yogurt
6 ounces feta cheese, crumbled
3 teaspoons dill
Salt and pepper to taste

Directions:

1. Heat the olive oil in a skillet and sauté the onions and garlic for a few minutes.

2. Stir in the spinach. Cover and cook for 5 minutes.

3. When the spinach is wilted, remove from heat.

4. Preheat the oven to 375 degrees F.

5. Mix together the cooked lentils and quinoa, the spinach, and tomatoes.

6. In another bowl, whisk the eggs and add the yogurt and feta. Season with the dill, salt, and pepper.

7. Stir the quinoa/lentil mixture into the egg mixture and mix thoroughly.

8. Transfer to a casserole dish and bake for 40 minutes.

Nutritional Information (Per Serving)
Calories: 480
Fat: 11.3 g
Sat Fat: 4.2 g
Carbohydrates: 69 g
Fiber: 20 g
Sugar: 4.2 g
Protein: 26.9 g
Sodium: 292 mg

Fully Loaded Baked Potato

Baked potato with sour cream? You can do better than that!

Makes 4 servings

Ingredients for the Potatoes:
4 russet potatoes
2 tablespoons olive oil
1 teaspoon oregano
Salt and pepper to taste

Ingredients for the Topping:
1 cup tzatziki sauce
½ cup parsley, chopped
1 tomato, diced
½ cup black olives, pitted and chopped
4 tablespoon crumbled feta cheese

Directions:
1. Preheat the oven to 375 degrees F.
2. Wash and dry the potatoes.
3. Coat potatoes with the olive oil and puncture them in a few places with a fork.
4. Place them on a baking sheet and bake for 1 hour. Check for doneness and transfer to a platter.
5. For the topping, cut the potatoes open and spoon the insides into a small bowl.
6. Mash the potato insides and add the olive oil, oregano, salt, and pepper. Mix well.
7. Stuff the potato skins with the mash.
8. Serve with tzatziki sauce.

Nutritional Information (Per Serving)
Calories: 258

Fat: 11.1 g
Sat Fat: 2.7 g
Carbohydrates: 36.2 g
Fiber: 6.3 g
Sugar: 3.3 g
Protein: 5.5 g

Stuffed Zucchini

Makes 6 servings

Ingredients:
6 medium zucchinis, halved lengthwise
2 potatoes, peeled and cubed
4 teaspoons olive oil
2½ cups onion, chopped
1 serrano pepper, minced
2 garlic cloves, minced
1½ tablespoons fresh ginger, minced
2 tablespoons chickpea flour
1 teaspoon ground coriander
¼ teaspoon ground cumin
1½ cups frozen green peas, thawed
2 tablespoons fresh cilantro, chopped
½ teaspoon salt
Black pepper to taste

Directions:
1. Preheat the oven to 375 degrees F.
2. With a scooper, scoop out the pulp from zucchini halves, leaving about ¼" thick shell.
3. In a shallow roasting pan, arrange the zucchini halves, cut side up. Sprinkle the zucchini halves with a little salt.
4. In a pan of boiling water, cook the potatoes for about 2 minutes. Drain well and set aside.

5. In a nonstick skillet, heat oil over medium-high heat. Add onion, serrano pepper, garlic, and ginger, and sauté for 3 minutes.

6. Reduce heat to medium low. Stir in chickpea flour and spices, and cook for about 5 minutes. Stir in cooked potatoes, green peas, and cilantro, and remove from heat.

7. With a paper towel, pat dry the zucchini halves. Stuff the zucchini halves evenly with the veggie mixture.

8. Lightly grease a baking dish. Arrange the zucchini halves in the baking dish.

9. Bake, covered for about 20 minutes.

Nutritional Information (Per Serving)
Calories: 150
Fat: 3.4 g
Sat Fat: 0.5 g
Carbohydrates: 25.2 g
Fiber: 5.8 g
Sugar: 3.1 g
Protein: 5.0 g
Sodium: 240 mg

Phyllo Spinach Pie

Tell the kids it's a pie, and they'll fight to eat spinach. Definitely a win-win.

Makes 8 servings

Ingredients for the Filling:

1 package frozen spinach, thawed and drained

½ cup parsley, chopped

1 onion, chopped

2 garlic cloves, minced

2 tablespoons olive oil

4 large eggs

10 ounces feta cheese, crumbled

2 teaspoons dill

Dash of black pepper

Ingredients for the Crust:

1 package phyllo dough, thawed

1 cup olive oil

Directions:

1. Preheat the oven to 325 degrees F.

2. Squeeze any liquid out of the spinach.

3. For the filling, mix all of the filling ingredients well.

4. For the crust, flatten the phyllo and cover them with a damp cloth.

5. Brush a baking dish with olive oil.

6. Place 2 phyllo sheets at the bottom of the baking dish. Sprinkle with olive oil.

7. Keep layering, using two-thirds of the phyllo sheets.

8. Top the phyllo sheets with the filling. Add more layers until you've used all the phyllo.

9. You need to drizzle each layer with olive oil, but be especially generous with the top layer.

10. Bake for 1 hour and cut the pie into squares.

Nutritional Information (Per Serving)
Calories: 421
Fat: 39.5 g
Sat Fat: 10.3 g
Carbohydrates: 9.9 g
Fiber: 1.4 g
Sugar: 2.4 g
Protein: 10.2 g
Sodium: 508 mg

Vegetarian Chili

Makes 8 servings

Ingredients:

2 cups onion, diced

1 cup celery, diced

1 cup bell pepper, diced

2 cloves garlic, minced

2 tablespoons water

2 jalapeño peppers, diced

4 cups crushed tomatoes, no salt added

2 cups canned pinto beans, drained and rinsed, no salt added

2 tablespoons cumin

1 tablespoon chipotle pepper

1 tablespoon black pepper

1 tablespoon balsamic vinegar

1 tablespoon oregano

Directions:

1. Add onion, celery, bell pepper, and garlic in 2 tablespoons of water in a stockpot over low heat. Cook until onions are translucent.

2. Add the rest of the ingredients. Cover and simmer for 1–2 hours, occasionally stirring.

3. If chili becomes too thick, thin it with water, adding small increments of water at a time.

Nutritional Information (Per Serving)
Calories: 115
Fat: 1.2 g
Sat Fat: 0.2 g
Carbohydrates: 22.9 g
Fiber: 6.7 g
Sugar: 0.8 g
Protein: 5.6 g
Sodium: 27.1 mg

CHAPTER FOUR

Poultry and Meats

Chicken Pasta

This chicken dish is brimming with Greek flavor. Healthy, delicious, and easy to prepare, it'll become a staple.

Makes 6 servings

Ingredients:
1 package pasta of your choice
¼ cup onions, diced
2 garlic gloves, minced
1 tablespoon olive oil
1 pound boneless chicken pieces
1 tomato, chopped
½ cup feta cheese
3 tablespoons lemon juice
2 tablespoons parsley, chopped
Salt and pepper to taste

Directions:
1. Cook the pasta according to directions.
2. Sauté the onion and garlic in the olive oil for 3 minutes in a skillet over medium-high heat.
3. Add the chicken pieces and cook for 7–8 minutes.
4. Lower the heat and add the remaining ingredients, including the pasta. Mix well.
5. Adjust seasoning and serve.

Nutritional Information (Per Serving)

Calories: 398
Fat: 8.3 g
Sat Fat: 2.3 g
Carbohydrates: 55 g
Fiber: 8.3 g
Sugar: 1.2 g
Protein: 29.9 g

Chicken Soup with Orzo

Makes 8 servings

Ingredients:

1½ pounds chicken meat, cubed

¼ teaspoon pepper

¼ teaspoon rosemary

¼ teaspoon thyme

¼ teaspoon cinnamon

1 tablespoon olive oil

4 scallions, chopped

1 garlic clove, minced

4 cups chicken broth

4 cups water

5 tablespoons chopped sun-dried tomatoes

5 tablespoons pitted and sliced black olives

2 cups orzo

2 tablespoons lemon juice

2 teaspoons chopped parsley

Directions:

1. Make a rub with all of the spices and season the chicken cubes.

2. Heat the olive oil in a large pot over medium-high heat and sauté the chicken for 3–4 minutes. Transfer the chicken to a platter.

3. In the same pot, sauté the scallion and garlic for one minute.

4. Add the broth, water, sun-dried tomatoes, olives and return the chicken to the pot.

5. Bring to a boil, then lower the heat to a simmer.

6. Let simmer for approximately 20 minutes.

7. Bring the broth back to a boil and add the orzo.

8. Cook for 15 more minutes.

9. And the parsley, lemon juice and stir.

Nutritional Information (Per Serving)
Calories: 311
Fat: 6.9 g
Sat Fat: 0.5 g
Carbohydrates: 34.1 g
Fiber: 1.9 g
Sugar: 3.1 g
Protein: 25.8 g
Sodium: 505 mg

Balsamic Chicken Wrap

Makes 2 servings

Ingredients:

2 whole grain flour tortillas

6 ounces cooked chicken which has been cooled

¼ cup balsamic vinegar

2 tablespoons spicy brown mustard

2 large leaves of romaine lettuce

¼ cup chopped red onion

Directions:

1. Marinate the cooked chicken in the balsamic vinegar and onion overnight in the refrigerator.

2. Spread one tablespoon of mustard on each tortilla and cover with a lettuce leaf.

3. Spoon the chicken mixture onto the lettuce and roll up the tortilla until you have a wrap.

Nutritional Information (Per Serving)
Calories: 287
Fat: 5.1 g
Sat Fat: 0.7 g
Carbohydrates: 26 g
Fiber: 5.3 g
Sugar: 1.9 g
Protein: 28.9 g
Sodium: 376 mg

Roasted Chicken

Cooking all of these ingredients together results in a symphony of subtle flavors.

Makes 6 servings

Ingredients:

2 tablespoon minced garlic

3 tablespoons olive oil

½ teaspoon salt

½ teaspoon thyme

½ teaspoon pepper

2 pounds chicken breast cut in pieces

¾ cup white wine

1 cup chicken broth

¾ cup red onion, sliced

1½ pounds small potatoes, halved

⅓ cup kalamata olives, pitted and halved

1½ cups tomatoes, diced

½ cup banana peppers, chopped

14 ounces artichoke hearts, quartered

2 ounces parmesan cheese, grated

1 tablespoon chopped basil

Directions:

1. Preheat the oven to 400 degrees F.

2. Combine 2 tablespoon of the oil, garlic, half the salt and half the pepper with the potatoes.

3. Bake for 30 minutes.

4. Heat the remaining olive oil in a Dutch oven over medium heat.

5. Season the chicken with the remaining salt and pepper.

6. Sauté the chicken for 5 minutes. To avoid overcrowding the pot, sauté in batches if needed. Set the chicken aside.

7. Add onion to the pot and sauté for 5 minutes. Pour in the wine and bring to a boil.

8. Cook for 2–3 minutes to reduce the liquid. Lower the heat and add the broth, chicken, potatoes, and olives.

9. Cook for 3 minutes.

10. Stir in the remaining ingredients, except the cheese, and cook for 5 more minutes.

11. Top with the parmesan and enjoy.

Nutritional Information (Per Serving)
Calories: 316
Fat: 12.6 g
Sat Fat: 3.2 g
Carbohydrates: 31.3 g
Fiber: 7.6 g
Sugar: 4.6 g
Protein: 17.2 g
Sodium: 573 mg

Baked Chicken Wings with Tzatziki Dipping Sauce

You don't need BBQ sauce for great wings. Try this refreshing tzatziki dip instead.

Makes 10 servings
Ingredients for the Marinade:
1 cup olive oil
Juice and zest from 2 lemons
6 crudely chopped garlic cloves
1 tablespoon paprika
1 tablespoon oregano
1 tablespoon salt
1 tablespoon pepper

Optional: 1 teaspoon cayenne pepper for extra heat.

Ingredients for the Wings:
3 pounds chicken wings
Lemon slices, crumbled feta cheese, and parsley as garnish

For the Tzatziki Dipping Sauce:
3 tablespoon olive oil
1 cup Greek yogurt
1 grated cucumber
2 minced garlic cloves
1 tablespoon lemon juice
2 tablespoon chopped mint
2 tablespoon chopped dill
Salt and pepper to taste

Directions:
1. In a bowl, mix the marinade ingredients. Marinate the wings overnight in the refrigerator.
2. Preheat the oven to 375 degrees F.
3. Place the chicken wings on a baking sheet and bake for 45 minutes.
4. Broil the wings for a few minutes to crisp them.
5. Make the dipping sauce while the chicken is baking. Whisk together the sauce ingredients and refrigerate.
6. Place the chicken wings on a platter. Garnish them and serve with the tzatziki dipping sauce.

Nutritional Information (Per Serving)
Calories: 499
Fat: 35.1 g
Sat Fat: 6.6 g
Carbohydrates: 4.7 g
Fiber: 1 g
Sugar: 2 g

Protein: 42.1 g

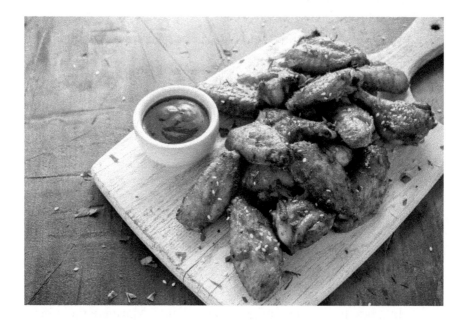

Balsamic Chicken and Beans

Makes 4 servings

Ingredients:

4 skinless, boneless chicken breasts

¼ cup balsamic vinegar

2 garlic cloves, minced

2 shallots, sliced

3 tablespoon extra-virgin olive oil

1 pound fresh green beans, trimmed

2 tablespoons red pepper flakes

Directions:

1. Combine 2 tablespoon of the olive oil with the balsamic vinegar, garlic, and shallots. Pour it over the chicken breasts and refrigerate overnight.

2. The next day, preheat the oven to 375 degrees F.

3. Take the chicken out of the marinade and arrange in a shallow baking pan. Discard the rest of the marinade.

3. Bake in the oven for 40 minutes.

4. While the chicken is cooking, bring a large pot of water to a boil. Place the green beans in the water and allow them to cook for five minutes and then drain.

5. Heat one tablespoon of olive oil in the pot and return the green beans after rinsing them. Toss with red pepper flakes.

Nutritional Information (Per Serving)
Calories: 433
Fat: 17.4 g
Sat Fat: 3.3 g
Carbohydrates: 12.9 g
Fiber: 4.6 g
Sugar: 3.1 g
Protein: 56.1 g
Sodium: 140 mg

Turkey Sausage and Peppers

Makes 4 servings

Ingredients:

4 turkey sausages, spicy or sweet

2 red bell peppers, chopped

2 green bell peppers, chopped

1 red onion, sliced

¼ cup olive oil

2 sprigs fresh rosemary

¼ cup fresh basil

4 cups brown rice, cooked

Directions:

1. Cook the sausages in the olive oil over medium-high heat until brown. Remove from heat and add the peppers and onions.

2. While the vegetables cook, slice the sausages into pieces. Add it back to the pan and cook everything together for 10 minutes.

3. Serve over rice and sprinkle with rosemary and basil.

Nutritional Information (Per Serving)

Calories: 374

Fat: 18.1 g

Sat Fat: 3 g

Carbohydrates: 46.8 g

Fiber: 4.5 g

Sugar: 7.3 g

Protein: 10.6 g

Sodium: 164 mg

Slow Cooker Mediterranean Short Ribs

These savory short ribs are a snap to make in the slow cooker. Serve with couscous.

Makes 8 servings

Ingredients:
3 pounds bone-in short ribs
2 cups tomatoes, chopped
3 garlic cloves, diced
½ cup dried apricots, halved
2 teaspoons grated ginger
2 teaspoons cumin
½ teaspoon cinnamon
Salt and pepper to taste

Directions:
1. Add all ingredients to a slow cooker and cook on low for 8 hours.
2. Prepare one package of couscous following package instructions, and serve with the ribs.

Nutritional Information (Per Serving)
Calories: 678
Fat: 61.8 g
Sat Fat: 27 g
Carbohydrates: 3.8 g
Fiber: 0.9 g
Sugar: 2.1 g
Protein: 24.7 g
Sodium: 86 mg

Grilled Steak

The Mediterranean diet doesn't include a lot of meat. But when it does, this is the way to do it.

Makes 2 servings

Ingredients:
2 steaks – your choice of cut
1 cup spinach, chopped
1 tablespoon olive oil
2 tablespoons red onions, diced
2 tablespoons feta cheese, crumbled
2 tablespoons panko breadcrumbs
1 tablespoon diced sun-dried tomato
Salt and pepper to taste

Directions:
1. Preheat grill to medium-high heat.
2. Use a skillet to sauté the onions in the olive oil for 5 minutes.
3. Add the remaining ingredients, except the steaks, and stir for 2 minutes. Take off the stove and let sit.
5. Grill the steaks to desired doneness.
6. Top each steak with the spinach mix. Cook in the broiler until the top turns brown.

Nutritional Information (Per Serving)
Calories: 531
Fat: 33.2 g
Sat Fat: 12.2 g
Carbohydrates: 37.8 g
Fiber: 1.6 g
Sugar: 0.9 g
Protein: 22.7 g
Sodium: 582 mg

Spicy Roasted Leg of Lamb

You want your leg of lamb roasted to a delicate pink, like a blush.

Makes 4 servings

Ingredients for the Lamb:

1 pound leg of lamb, with bone

Salt and pepper to taste

3 tablespoons olive oil

5 garlic cloves, sliced

2 cups water

4 potatoes, cubed

1 onion, roughly chopped

1 teaspoon garlic powder

Ingredients for the Lamb Spice Rub:

15 garlic cloves, peeled

3 tablespoons oregano

2 tablespoons mint

1 tablespoon paprika

½ cup olive oil

¼ cup lemon juice

Directions:

1. Let the lamb sit at room temperature for an hour.

2. While you wait, put all of the spice rub ingredients in a food processor and blend. Refrigerate the rub.

3. Using a sharp knife, make a few cuts in the lamb. Season with salt and pepper.

4. Place on a roasting pan.

5. Heat the broiler and broil for 5 minutes on each side so the whole thing is seared.

6. Place the lamb on the counter and set the oven temperature to 375 degrees F.

7. Let the lamb cool, then fill the cuts with the garlic slices and cover with the spice rub.

8. Add 2 cups of water to the roasting pan.

9. Sprinkle the potatoes and onions with the garlic powder, salt, and pepper. Arrange them around the leg of lamb.

10. Loosely cover the roasting pan with aluminum foil and place it back in the oven.

11. Roast the lamb for 1 hour.

12. Discard the foil and roast for 15 more minutes.

13. Let the leg of lamb sit for 20 minutes before serving.

Nutritional Information (Per Serving)
Calories: 504
Fat: 19.9 g
Sat Fat: 4.8 g
Carbohydrates: 45.2 g
Fiber: 8.5 g
Sugar: 4.6 g
Protein: 37.6 g
Sodium: 111 mg

CHAPTER FIVE

Fish and Seafood

Spicy Shrimp Salad

Shrimp is a great protein source, especially when you grow tired of chicken and eggs. This shrimp salad is tangy and if you don't like it on the cukes, put it on some whole grain bread or in a high fiber tortilla.

Makes 2 servings

Ingredients:

½ pound salad shrimp, chopped

2 stalks celery, chopped

¼ cup red onion, diced

1 teaspoon black pepper

1 teaspoon red pepper

1 tablespoon lemon juice

Dash of cayenne pepper

1 tablespoon olive oil

2 cucumbers, sliced thick

Directions:

1. Combine the shrimp, celery, and onion in a bowl and mix together.

2. In a separate bowl, whisk the oil and the lemon juice, then add red pepper, black pepper, and cayenne pepper. Pour over the shrimp and mix.

3. Serve on slices of thickly cut cucumber pieces.

Nutritional Information (Per Serving)

Calories: 245
Fat: 9 g
Sat Fat: 1.2 g
Carbohydrates: 18.2 g
Fiber: 3.2 g
Sugar: 9.1 g
Protein: 27.3 g
Sodium: 280 mg

Salmon Spinach Salad

Mediterraneans love spinach and fresh fish. You'll love this salad.

Makes 2 servings

Ingredients:

1 6-ounce piece of salmon, cooked and chopped into pieces

8 ounces of spinach leaves, washed and chopped

1 Clementine orange, peeled with fibers removed

¼ cup red onion, sliced thin

¼ cup walnuts, chopped

2 ounces feta cheese, crumbled

¼ cup raisins

3 tablespoons olive oil

2 tablespoons red wine vinegar

Directions:

1. Toss the spinach leaves with the orange segments, onion, walnuts, cheese, and raisins.

2. Add the salmon pieces and mix together.

3. Cover with olive oil and vinegar.

Nutritional Information (Per Serving)

Calories: 571

Fat: 42.1 g

Sat Fat: 8.6 g

Carbohydrates: 27.1 g

Fiber: 5.2 g

Sugar: 16.6 g

Protein: 28.6 g

Sodium: 447 mg

Tuna Salad with Capers

Capers are a huge part of the Mediterranean diet, and most people either love or hate their strong, daring taste. Try them with tuna.

Makes 2 servings

Ingredients:

1 can tuna

6 ounces lettuce

1 medium tomato, sliced

¼ cup olives, chopped

½ red bell pepper, sliced

½ cup cucumber, chopped

¼ cup capers, drained and rinsed

2 tablespoons olive oil

2 tablespoons balsamic vinegar

Directions:

1. Chop the lettuce and place it in a medium bowl. Add the tomato, olives, pepper, and cucumber.

2. Toss together with the olive oil and vinegar.

3. Top the salad with the tuna and then the capers.

Nutritional Information (Per Serving)

Calories: 348

Fat: 23.5 g

Sat Fat: 3.8 g

Carbohydrates: 10.2 g

Fiber: 2.9 g

Sugar: 4.5 g

Protein: 25.6 g

Sodium: 710 mg

Pasta with Shrimp

This savory dish is definitely company-worthy.

Makes 4 servings

Ingredients:

4 cups prepared linguini
1 tablespoon olive oil
2 garlic cloves, minced
1 pound shrimp, peeled and deveined
1½ cups tomato, diced
4 tablespoons chopped basil
6 tablespoons diced kalamata olives
2 tablespoons capers
Dash of ground pepper
2 ounces feta cheese, crumbled

Directions:

1. Sauté the garlic in the olive oil for one minute.
2. Stir in the shrimp and sauté for another minute.
3. Mix in the diced tomato and chopped basil and let simmer for 4 minutes.
4. Add the capers, olives, and pepper.
5. Toss the shrimp mixture with the prepared pasta.
6. Sprinkle the feta cheese on top of the dish.

Nutritional Information (Per Serving)
Calories: 475
Fat: 11.4 g
Sat Fat: 3.5 g
Carbohydrates: 54.5 g
Fiber: 4.6 g
Sugar: 9.1 g
Protein: 37.4 g
Sodium: 385 mg

Lemon Pepper Cod with Chickpeas

Makes 4 servings

Ingredients:

4 pieces of fresh cod (about 1½ pounds total)

1 lemon, juiced

1 lemon, sliced

1 tablespoon black pepper

1 tablespoon white pepper

¼ cup olive oil plus 1 tablespoon

1 can chickpeas, drained and rinsed

12 ounces fresh spinach

Directions:

1. Preheat the oven to 375 degrees F.

2. Place the slices of lemon on the bottom of a baking pan, and layer the fish on top of them. Drizzle half of the ¼ cup olive oil onto the fish and then add the lemon juice.

3. Sprinkle with both peppers and cook until the fish begins to flake, about 15–20 minutes.

4. Sauté the spinach in the remaining ¼ cup of olive oil until it wilts and gets hot. Cook the chickpeas in a small saucepan.

5. When the fish is ready to come out, plate it with the chickpeas and spinach.

6. Cover everything with the remaining olive oil.

Nutritional Information (Per Serving)
Calories: 458
Fat: 22 g
Sat Fat: 2.9 g
Carbohydrates: 40 g
Fiber: 12.2 g
Sugar: 6.5 g
Protein: 28.4 g
Sodium: 81 mg

Mediterranean Baked Salmon

This dish combines the goodness of salmon with green salad ingredients. What could be better?

Makes 8 servings

Ingredients:

8 salmon fillets
¼ cup olive oil
4 tomatoes, diced
⅓ cup feta cheese, crumbled
6 tablespoons diced red onion
1 tablespoon chopped basil
2 tablespoons lemon juice

Directions:

1. Preheat the oven to 350 degrees F.
2. Brush the salmon with olive oil and place in a baking dish.
3. Top the fillets with the remaining ingredients and bake for 20 minutes. The salmon should be flaky.

Nutritional Information (Per Serving)
Calories: 321
Fat: 18.8 g
Sat Fat: 3.5 g
Carbohydrates: 3.4 g
Fiber: 0.9 g
Sugar: 2.3 g
Protein: 36.1 g
Sodium: 152 mg

Pepper Tilapia with Spinach

Makes 4 servings

Ingredients:

4 tilapia filets, 8 ounces each

4 cups fresh spinach

1 red onion, sliced

3 garlic cloves, minced

2 tablespoons extra virgin olive oil

3 lemons

1 tablespoon ground black pepper

1 tablespoon ground white pepper

1 tablespoon crushed red pepper

Directions:

1. Preheat the oven to 350 degrees F.

2. Place the fish in a shallow baking dish and juice two of the lemons.

3. Cover the fish in the lemon juice and then sprinkle the three types of pepper over the fish.

4. Slice the remaining lemon and cover the fish. Bake in the oven for 20 minutes.

5. While the fish cooks, sauté the garlic and onion in the olive oil. Add the spinach.

6. Serve the fish on top of the spinach.

Nutritional Information (Per Serving)
Calories: 323
Fat: 11.5 g
Sat Fat: 2.1 g
Carbohydrates: 10.3 g
Fiber: 2.6 g
Sugar: 1.1 g
Protein: 50.0 g
Sodium: 145 mg

Baked Snapper with Olives

Cooking snapper in foil intensifies the flavor. To enjoy all of the juices, serve the snapper with rice or crusty bread.

Makes 2 servings

Ingredients:

2 tomatoes, chopped

1 shallot, diced

2 tablespoons olive oil

1 teaspoon thyme

2 snapper fillets

Salt and pepper to taste

Directions:

1. Preheat the oven to 450 degrees F.

2. Mix the tomatoes and thyme in a bowl. Add the shallots and 1 tablespoon of oil.

3. Cut an 18" piece of aluminum foil and add the remaining oil in the middle of the foil.

4. Place the fillets on top of the oil, then spoon the tomatoes on top. Sprinkle with salt and pepper.

5. Close the foil packet and tighten the edges.

6. Place the foil packet on a baking dish and bake for 15–20 minutes, until the fish is flaky.

7. Let the fish sit for a few minutes. Carefully open the foil to avoid burning yourself and to not lose any of the juices.

8. Serve with rice or crusty bread.

Nutritional Information (Per Serving)

Calories: 298

Fat: 16 g

Sat Fat: 2 g

Carbohydrates: 5.9 g

Fiber: 1.7 g

Sugar: 3.2 g
Protein: 33.2 g

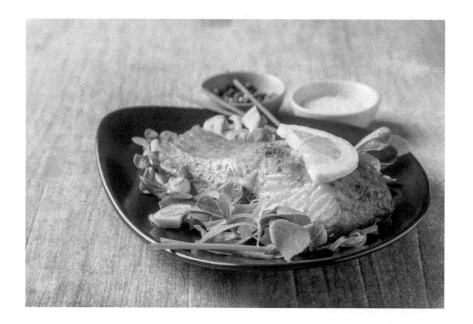

CHAPTER SIX

Snacks

Grilled Figs and Goat Cheese

We should be eating more fresh figs. They are so sweet, smooth, chewy, and just about perfect. On its own, the fig is wonderful. With the goat cheese, it's heavenly.

Makes 5 servings

Ingredients:

10 fresh figs

¾ cup goat cheese, softened

10 grape leaves

¼ cup honey

Directions:

1. Preheat grill to medium heat.

2. Make a cut in the bottom of the figs.

3. Place the goat cheese in a pastry bag and pipe the cheese into the figs through the cut.

4. Wrap each fig with a grape leaf and place 3–4 figs on a skewer.

5. Grill for about 3 minutes. Turn the skewer around once.

6. Drizzle with the honey

Nutritional Information (Per Serving)

Calories: 176

Fat: 2.7 g

Sat Fat: 1.7 g

Carbohydrates: 38.3 g

Fiber: 3.8 g

Sugar: 32.2 g

Protein: 3.4 g
Sodium: 46 mg

Caprese Kebobs

Few things are as abundant in the Mediterranean as tomatoes. Put them to good use with this simple snack.

Makes 3 servings
Ingredients:
15 grape tomatoes
½ cup mozzarella cheese, cut into cubes
3 fresh basil leaves
1 tablespoon olive oil
1 tablespoon balsamic vinegar
Sprinkle of sea salt
Black pepper
3 kebab spears

Directions:
1. Divide the grape tomatoes and the mozzarella cubes into three piles. Place a tomato, then a chunk of cheese on each spear until you have used up your ingredients.

2. One basil leaf should also go on each kebob.

3. Drizzle with oil and vinegar and sprinkle with salt and pepper.

Nutritional Information (Per Serving)
Calories: 165
Fat: 6.7 g
Sat Fat: 1.3 g
Carbohydrates: 24.2 g
Fiber: 7.4 g
Sugar: 16.2 g

Protein: 6.8 g
Sodium: 59 mg

Spicy Olives

You'll love munching on these spiced olives.

Makes 8 servings

Ingredients:
2 teaspoons coriander seeds
½ cup olive oil
4 pieces orange zest
2 teaspoons diced garlic clove
2 cups olives
1 tablespoon ouzo

Directions:
1. Crush the coriander seeds with a mortar and pestle.
2. Place them in a small pan and stir while cooking for one minute.
3. Add the olive oil and the rest of the spices and stir for another minute.
4. Add the olives and the ouzo and cook until the olives are warmed.
5. Strain the mixture into a bowl.
6. If desired, use some crusty bread to dip in the oil.

Nutritional Information (Per Serving)
Calories: 148
Fat: 16.2 g
Sat Fat: 2.3 g
Carbohydrates: 2.4 g
Fiber: 1.1 g
Sugar: 0 g
Protein: 0.3 g

Sodium: 293 mg

Marinated Olives & Feta Cheese

Olives and feta cheese are truly the best food marriage.

Makes 8 servings

Ingredients:

2 cups kalamata olives

½ cup feta cheese, cubed

4 tablespoons olive oil

3 tablespoons lemon juice

3 garlic cloves, minced

2 teaspoons rosemary

¼ teaspoon black pepper

Directions:

1. Combine all the ingredients in a bowl and refrigerate for at least 1 hour.

Nutritional Information (Per Serving)

Calories: 128

Fat: 12.7 g

Sat Fat: 3 g

Carbohydrates: 3.2 g

Fiber: 1.3 g

Sugar: 0.5 g

Protein: 1.8 g

Sodium: 399 mg

Roasted Eggplant Dip

Be sure to get eggplants when they're in season. They make a great healthy snack.

Makes 4 servings

Ingredients:
1 eggplant
¼ cup olive oil
½ cup feta cheese
½ cup red onion, diced
2 tablespoons lemon juice
1 bell pepper, diced
1 tablespoon chopped basil
Salt and pepper to taste

Directions:
1. Preheat the broiler. The rack should be 6–7 inches from the heat.

2. Cover a baking pan with aluminum foil and place the eggplant on top.

3. Broil for about 18–20 minutes, turning it 3 times. Let the eggplant cool

4. Place the lemon juice in a small bowl.

5. Cut the eggplant open and spoon the flesh out. Add flesh to the lemon juice and coat. Pour in the olive oil and stir.

6. Add the remaining ingredients and blend well.

7. Serve with fresh vegetables or pita chips.

Nutritional Information (Per Serving)
Calories: 203
Fat: 17 g
Sat Fat: 4.7 g
Carbohydrates: 11.3 g
Fiber: 4.8 g

Sugar: 6.5 g
Protein: 4.3 g

Basic Hummus

This flavorful hummus is so easy to prepare.

Makes 4 servings

Ingredients:

1 can garbanzo beans

2 ounces jalapeno pepper, sliced

2 garlic cloves, minced

½ teaspoon cumin

2 tablespoons lemon juice

Directions:

1. Combine all of the ingredients in a blender and blend until smooth.

Nutritional Information (Per Serving)

Calories: 81

Fat: 0.9 g

Sat Fat: 0.1 g

Carbohydrates: 15.2 g

Fiber: 3.1 g

Sugar: 0.7 g

Protein: 3.4 g

Sodium: 182 mg

Feta Hummus

Store-bought hummus doesn't even come close. Keep this nutty dip handy for when you feel like snacking on cucumbers, carrots, or pita.

Makes 12 servings

Ingredients:
1½ cups dried chickpeas
1 teaspoon baking soda
3 garlic cloves, diced
½ cup tahini
⅓ cup lemon juice (adjust for taste)
1 teaspoon salt
⅓ cup olive oil
⅓ cup feta cheese, crumbled
2 tablespoons chopped parsley

Directions:
1. Place the chickpeas in a bowl of water and refrigerate overnight.

2. In a large pot, combine the chickpeas and baking soda and cook for 3 minutes while stirring.

3. Pour in 8 cups of water and bring to a boil.

4. Lower the heat and add the garlic. Let simmer for about 1 hour.

5. Drain all of the water except for ¼ cup.

6. Place the chickpeas in a bowl filled with water and agitate to help loosen their skins. Use a slotted spoon to discard skins.

7. Drain the chickpeas and place them in a food processor. Purée until smooth.

8. While pureeing, add in the ¼ cup reserved water, tahini, lemon juice, and salt.

9. Once blended transfer the hummus to a bowl and refrigerate for one hour.

10. When you are ready to use the hummus, adjust the seasoning and drizzle with the oil.

11. Top with the feta and parsley.

Nutritional Information (Per Serving)
Calories: 212
Fat: 13.4 g
Sat Fat: 2.4 g
Carbohydrates: 17.9 g
Fiber: 5.4 g
Sugar: 3.1 g
Protein: 7.2 g
Sodium: 364 mg

Spiced Nuts

If you're someone who needs a crunch with your snacking habit, these hot and tasty nuts will satisfy your craving.

Makes 20 servings

Ingredients:

1 cup almonds

1 cup walnuts

1 cup cashews

1 cup peanuts

¼ teaspoon cayenne pepper

½ teaspoon red pepper flakes

¼ teaspoon chili powder

1 tablespoon olive oil

½ cup raisins

Directions:

1. Preheat the oven to 375 degrees F.

2. In a bowl, mix all the nuts with the olive oil and the spices. Toss with your hands until everything is coated.

3. Layer the nuts onto a baking sheet and cook in the oven for 20–30 minutes.

4. Remove the nuts and allow them to cool for about 5 minutes. Then, put them back into the bowl and toss with the raisins.

Nutritional Information (Per Serving)

Calories: 164

Fat: 13.6 g

Sat Fat: 1.6 g

Carbohydrates: 8 g

Fiber: 2 g

Sugar: 3.1 g

Protein: 5.6 g

Sodium: 3 mg

Fruity Nut Bars

Makes 24 bars

Ingredients:

½ cup quinoa flour

½ cup oats

¼ cup flax meal

¼ cup wheat germ

¼ cup chopped almonds

¼ cup dried apricots

¼ cup dried figs

¼ cup honey

2 tablespoons cornstarch

Directions:

1. Preheat the oven to 300 degrees F.

2. In a large bowl, combine all ingredients and mix thoroughly.

3. Spread mixture in a half an inch-thick layer in a parchment-lined sheet pan and bake for 20 minutes.

4. Let cool and cut.

Nutritional Information (Per Bar)

Calories: 53.8

Fat: 1.3 g

Sat Fat: 0.1 g

Carbohydrates: 9.7 g

Fiber: 1.4 g

Sugar: 4.7 g

Protein: 1.4 g

Sodium: 1.4 mg

Tomato Sandwiches with Basil

Fresh tomatoes are bursting with flavor.

Makes 2 servings

Ingredients:

2 slices whole-wheat bread

4 teaspoons mashed avocado

2 tomato slices

2 teaspoons chopped basil

Salt and pepper to taste

Direction:

1. Cut the bread into discs the size of the tomato slices. (Use a biscuit cutter)

2. Distribute the avocado equally onto each bread round.

3. Top with the tomatoes and basil. Season according to taste.

Nutritional Information (Per Serving)

Calories: 175

Fat: 10.8 g

Sat Fat: 2.3 g

Carbohydrates: 16.5 g

Fiber: 5.5 g

Sugar: 2.2 g

Protein: 4.7 g

Date Wraps

Makes 5 servings
Ingredients:
10 thin slices of prosciutto
10 dates, pitted
Pepper to taste

Directions:
1. Encase each date with 1 slice of prosciutto.
2. Sprinkle with pepper.

Nutritional Information (Per Serving)
Calories: 72
Fat: 1.5 g
Sat Fat: 0.6 g
Carbohydrates: 12.5 g
Fiber: 1.3 g
Sugar: 10.5 g
Protein: 3.3 g
Sodium: 186 mg

CHAPTER SEVEN

Dessert

Galatopita

This is a simple pudding that makes a perfect weeknight dessert.

Makes 10 servings
Ingredients:
4½ cups milk
1 cup semolina flour
½ cup honey
5 eggs
Olive oil cooking spray
Dash of vanilla

Directions:
1. Preheat oven to 375 degrees F.
2. Whisk the eggs.
3. Place all the ingredients in a pan.
4. Cook the pudding over medium heat while continuously stirring until the custard is thick.
5. Grease a baking pan with cooking spray and pour in the custard.
6. Bake for about an hour.
7. Turn off the heat and let the pudding cool for another 15 minutes.

Nutritional Information (Per Serving)
Calories: 198
Fat: 4.6 g
Sat Fat: 2.1 g

Carbohydrates: 31.7 g
Fiber: 0.7 g
Sugar: 19 g
Protein: 8.5 g
Sodium: 83 mg

Apples with Parmesan

The tartness of the apples pairs nicely with the sharp bite of the parmesan in this Mediterranean treat.

Makes 4 servings

Ingredients:

4 green apples, cored and sliced

4 ounces parmesan cheese, shaved thin

2 tablespoons honey

Directions:

1. Arrange the apple slices on a plate and cover them with the thin shavings of parmesan.

2. Drizzle with honey and serve.

Nutritional Information (Per Serving)

Calories: 201
Fat: 6 g
Sat Fat: 4 g
Carbohydrates: 31.4 g
Fiber: 4.9 g
Sugar: 25.4 g
Protein: 9 g
Sodium: 260 mg

Pudding Parfait

Makes 4 servings

Ingredients:

1 package Jell-O sugar-free, fat-free instant chocolate pudding

2 cups skim milk

½ cup sliced strawberries

1 banana, sliced

½ cup blueberries

Directions:

1. In a large bowl, whisk the instant pudding mix together with cold milk.

2. Once it's combined, cover the pudding and refrigerate. It should set within 30 minutes.

3. Set out four dessert cups. On the bottom of each one, place a few berries. Cover with pudding, and then place a layer of bananas in the cups. Add more pudding, and place a layer of berries.

4. Do this until all the pudding and fruit are evenly divided.

Nutritional Information (Per Serving)
Calories: 96
Fat: 0.2 g
Sat Fat: 0 g
Carbohydrates: 18.8 g
Fiber: 1.8 g
Sugar: 12.3 g
Protein: 4.6 g
Sodium: 143 mg

Fruit and Yogurt Lasagna

This is a great dessert and if you have a little bit of fruit and yogurt leftover, it also makes a great snack in the middle of the morning when you're not sure you'll make it to lunch.

Makes 4 servings
Ingredients:
4 dessert cups
1 cup blueberries
1 cup strawberries
1 cup blackberries
2 cups plain Greek yogurt
¼ cup crushed walnuts

Directions:
1. Place a scoop of yogurt in each cup. Then, create layers of fruit and yogurt.

2. First do the strawberries and then more yogurt. Then, do the blueberries followed by yogurt and then the blackberries.

3. Top each dessert cup with yogurt and sprinkle with crushed walnuts.

Nutritional Information (Per Serving)
Calories: 116
Fat: 3.2 g
Sat Fat: 1.4 g
Carbohydrates: 14.7 g
Fiber: 3.7 g
Sugar: 10.1 g
Protein: 8.8 g
Sodium: 26 mg

Banana Balls

These make a great dessert or snack. They're fast and easy to make, and you get a chocolate snack without overindulging. This isn't an everyday treat, but something you can enjoy while following the Mediterranean eating plan.

Makes 8 servings

Ingredients:

3 ripe bananas

½ cup peanut butter

¼ cup dark chocolate chips

¼ cup whole grain oats

Directions:

1. Preheat the oven to 350 degrees F.

2. Mash the bananas until they're smooth. Stir in the peanut butter, chocolate chips and oats.

3. Roll into balls and place on a baking sheet.

4. Bake for 20 minutes, until the outside starts to brown.

Nutritional Information (Per Serving)

Calories: 162

Fat: 9.5 g

Sat Fat: 2.4 g

Carbohydrates: 17.6 g

Fiber: 2.4 g

Sugar: 9 g

Protein: 5.1 g

Sodium: 75 mg

Chocolate Hazelnut Baklava

Makes 20 servings

Ingredients for the Pastry:

2 cups hazelnuts

5 ounces semisweet chocolate, chopped

3 tablespoons honey

½ teaspoon cinnamon

½ pound phyllo dough

½ cup olive oil

Ingredients for the Syrup:

5 tablespoons water

1 cup honey

1¼ teaspoons instant espresso coffee

2 tablespoons Kahlua liqueur

Directions:

1. Preheat the oven to 350 degrees F.

2. Finely grind the hazelnuts, chocolate, cinnamon, and honey in a food processor. Set aside.

3. Roll out the phyllo dough and cut into 9" x 9" squares. Place a damp towel over the phyllo dough.

4. Grease a square 9" baking pan. Lay a phyllo square in the pan and brush with olive oil.

5. Keep adding 6 more layers of phyllo squares, brushing each layer with the oil.

6. Transfer the ground hazelnut/chocolate mix over the phyllo.

7. Layer and oil the remaining phyllo squares.

8. Using a sharp knife, cut the phyllo into 9 squares. Halve each of the squares to create triangles.

9. Bake for 35 minutes and let cool.

10. To make the syrup, place all ingredients, except the Kahlua, in a pan and bring to a boil. Reduce heat and let simmer until the syrup thickens.

11. Remove from heat and stir in the Kahlua. Pour the hot syrup over the baklava.

12. Let sit for 5–6 hours before serving.

Nutritional Information (Per Serving)
Calories: 226
Fat: 12.4 g
Sat Fat: 2.5 g
Carbohydrates: 30 g
Fiber: 1.4 g
Sugar: 22.4 g
Protein: 2.3 g
Sodium: 56 mg

CHAPTER EIGHT

Mediterranean Diet Instant Pot Recipes

Good Morning Quinoa

Makes 6 servings

Ingredients:

1½ cups quinoa, rinsed and drained

2¼ cups water

2 tablespoons maple syrup

½ teaspoon vanilla

¼ teaspoon ground cinnamon

Salt   to   taste

Directions:

1. Add all the ingredients to your Instant Pot.

2. Close the lid, choose MANUAL, and cook at high pressure for 1 minute.

3. When the cooking is complete, do a natural pressure release for 10 minutes. Quick release the remaining pressure.

4. Fluff the quinoa with fork. Serve with sliced almonds or berries.

Nutritional Information (Per Serving)
Calories: 175
Fat: 2.6 g
Sat Fat: 0.3 g
Carbohydrates: 31.9 g
Fiber: 3 g
Sugar: 4 g
Protein: 6 g

Crustless Seafood Quiche

Makes 6 servings

Ingredients:

4 large eggs

1 cup half and half

1 teaspoon salt

1 teaspoon pepper

1 teaspoon smoked paprika

1 teaspoon Herbs de Provence

1 cup shredded parmesan cheese

1 cup green onions, chopped

8 ounces crab meat

8 ounces raw shrimp, chopped

Directions:

1. Using a large bowl, whisk together the eggs and half and half.

2. Add salt, pepper and paprika, Herbs de Provence, and shredded cheese. Mix well with fork.

3. Stir in green onions.

4. Add seafood and mix well.

5. Place a springform pan on a sheet of aluminum foil larger than the pan. Crimp foil around bottom of pan. Pour in egg mixture then cover loosely with foil.

6. Place a trivet inside the Instant Pot and fill with 1½ cups of water.

7. Place the covered springform pan on the trivet.

8. Close the lid and cook at high pressure for 30 minutes.

9. When the cooking is complete, do a natural pressure release for 10 minutes. Quick release the remaining pressure.

10. Carefully lift out the springform pan from the Instant Pot and let cool.

11. Use a knife to gently loosen the quiche from the pan. Remove the outer ring of the pan. Serve quiche warm or at room temperature.

Nutritional Information (Per Serving)
Calories: 228
Fat: 12.5 g
Sat Fat: 6 g
Carbohydrates: 5.2 g
Fiber: 0.7 g
Sugar: 0.8 g
Protein: 22.9 g
Sodium: 882 mg

Quick Vegetable Curry

Makes 6 servings
Ingredients:
1 tablespoon olive oil
1 large onion, diced
1 teaspoon mustard seed
½ teaspoon salt
4 garlic cloves, chopped
2 teaspoons curry powder
1 teaspoon ginger root, grated
¼ teaspoon cayenne pepper
1 cup vegetable broth
14 ounces coconut milk
1 large delicata squash, chopped
1 red bell pepper, diced
4 cups kale, chopped
14 ounces chickpeas, rinsed and drained
Chopped fresh cilantro for garnish

Directions:

1. Set the Instant Pot to SAUTÉ and heat the olive oil.

2. Add onion, mustard seeds, and salt, browning the onion slightly or about 4 minutes.

3. Add garlic, curry, ginger, and cayenne. Stir well until the mixture is fragrant and darkening slightly, about a minute and a half.

4. Add broth and coconut milk. Mix well.

5. Add squash, bell pepper, kale, and chickpeas. Stir to mix well.

6. Press CANCEL, close the lid, and cook at high pressure for 3 minutes.

7. When the cooking is complete, do a natural pressure release.

8. Garnish with chopped cilantro and serve.

Nutritional Information (Per Serving)
Calories: 474
Fat: 22.8 g
Sat Fat: 14.8 g
Carbohydrates: 55.6 g
Fiber: 15.4 g
Sugar: 12.5 g
Protein: 17.9 g
Sodium: 374 mg

Chipotle Black Beans

Makes 4 servings

Ingredients:

1 tablespoon olive oil

½ onion, diced

3 garlic cloves, minced

3 cups water

1 cup dried black beans, rinsed

2 teaspoon cumin

1 teaspoon smoked paprika

½ teaspoon chipotle powder

1 teaspoon salt

Directions:

1. Set the Instant Pot to SAUTÉ and heat the olive oil.

2. Add onion and garlic. Cook until onion turns clear, stirring frequently.

3. Add water, beans, and seasonings. Stir to mix well.

4. Press CANCEL, close the lid, and cook at high pressure for 35 minutes.

5. When the cooking is complete, do a natural pressure release.

Nutritional Information (Per Serving)
Calories: 210
Fat: 4.5 g
Sat Fat: 0.7 g
Carbohydrates: 33 g
Fiber: 8 g
Sugar: 1.7 g
Protein: 11 g
Sodium: 592 mg

Spiced Okra

Makes 4 servings

Ingredients:

2 tablespoons olive oil

6 garlic cloves, chopped

1 teaspoon cumin seeds

2 medium onions, sliced

2 medium tomatoes, chopped

2 pounds okra, cut into 1-inch pieces

½ cup vegetable broth

1 teaspoon ground coriander

½ teaspoon red chili powder

½ teaspoon ground turmeric

Salt and pepper to taste

Directions:

1. Place the oil in the Instant Pot and select SAUTÉ. Add the garlic and cumin seeds and cook for 1 minute.

2. Add the onion and cook for 4 minutes.

3. Add the remaining ingredients and cook for 1 more minute.

4. Press CANCEL and stir well.

5. Secure the lid and cook at high pressure for 2 minutes.

6. When the cooking is complete, do a quick pressure release.

7. Serve hot.

Nutritional Information (Per Serving)
Calories: 199
Fat: 8 g
Sat Fat: 1.2 g
Carbohydrates: 26.6 g
Fiber: 9.5 g
Sugar: 7.5 g
Protein: 6.6 g

Spinach with Tomatoes

Makes 4 servings

Ingredients:

2 tablespoons olive oil

2 small onions, chopped

2 teaspoons garlic, minced

10 cups fresh spinach, chopped

1 cup tomatoes, chopped

½ cup tomato puree

1½ cups vegetable broth

1 tablespoon fresh lemon juice

½ teaspoon red pepper flakes, crushed

Salt and pepper to taste

Directions:

1. Place the oil in the Instant Pot and select SAUTÉ. Add the onion and cook for about 3 minutes.

2. Add the garlic and red pepper flakes and cook for 1 minute.

3. Add spinach and cook for 2 minutes.

4. Press the CANCEL button and stir in the remaining ingredients.

5. Secure the lid and cook at high pressure for 6 minutes.

6. When the cooking is complete, carefully do a quick pressure release.

7. Serve warm.

Nutritional Information (Per Serving)

Calories: 168

Fat: 9.5 g

Sat Fat: 1.6 g

Carbohydrates: 12.5 g

Fiber: 3.6 g

Sugar: 5.6 g

Protein: 10.3 g

Lemon Garlic Chicken

Makes 4 servings

Ingredients:

6 boneless, skinless chicken thighs

½ teaspoon garlic powder

½ teaspoon smoked paprika

4 tablespoons olive oil, divided

½ small onion, chopped

4 garlic cloves, minced

3 teaspoon Italian seasoning

½ cup low sodium chicken broth

2 tablespoons light cream

Zest of half a lemon

Juice of 1 lemon

Chopped Italian parsley for garnish

Salt and pepper to taste

Directions:

1. In a large bowl, mix chicken with salt, pepper, garlic powder, and paprika.

2. Set the Instant Pot to SAUTÉ and heat 2 tablespoons olive oil.

3. Place chicken in the pot and cook on each side for 2–3 minutes or until browned. Remove chicken and set aside.

4. Heat 2 tablespoons olive oil in the pot and add onion and garlic. After a couple of minutes, add lemon juice to deglaze.

5. Add Italian seasoning, lemon zest, and chicken broth.

6. Return the chicken to the Instant Pot, press CANCEL, close the lid, and cook at high pressure for 12 minutes sealing.

7. When the cooking is complete, use a natural pressure release.

8. Remove chicken from the pot and set aside on a large serving plate.

9. Add light cream to the cooking liquid, stirring well. Thicker sauce can be created by adding some cornstarch, about ½ teaspoon.

10. Turn off Instant Pot, then reintroduce chicken to the pot to coat with sauce thoroughly.

11. Garnish with chopped parsley and serve.

Nutritional Information (Per Serving)
Calories: 284
Fat: 23.4 g
Sat Fat: 5.1 g
Carbohydrates: 2.9 g
Fiber: 0.4 g
Sugar: 0.9 g
Protein: 19.8 g

Cilantro Lime Drumsticks

Makes 3 servings

Ingredients:

1 tablespoon olive oil

6 chicken drumsticks

4 cloves garlic, minced

1 teaspoon red pepper, crushed

1 teaspoon cayenne pepper

½ teaspoon salt

Juice of 1 lime

½ cup chicken broth

2 tablespoons cilantro, chopped

Directions:

1. Set the Instant Pot to SAUTÉ and add the olive oil.

2. When the oil is hot, add drumsticks, garlic, red pepper, cayenne pepper, and salt. Use tongs to brown drumsticks on each side, for 2 minutes each.

3. Add lime juice and chicken broth. Mix well

4. Press CANCEL, close the lid, and cook at high pressure for 10 minutes.

5. When the cooking is complete, use a natural pressure release.

6. Garnish with cilantro and serve.

Nutritional Information (Per Serving)

Calories: 226

Fat: 10.4 g

Sat Fat: 2.1 g

Carbohydrates: 6.1 g

Fiber: 0.9 g

Sugar: 2.5 g

Protein: 26.9 g

Sodium: 591 mg

Mediterranean Beef

Makes 4 servings

Ingredients:

2 pounds chuck roast, trimmed

2 tablespoons whole wheat flour

½ teaspoon salt

1 teaspoon black pepper

½ teaspoon oregano

2 tablespoons olive oil

1 large onion, chopped

4 shallots, sliced

1 garlic clove, minced

½ cup beef broth

¼ cup red wine

¼ cup balsamic vinegar

½ cup dates, pitted and chopped

Directions:

1. Whisk flour, salt, pepper, and oregano in a bowl.

2. Slicing against the grain, chop beef into two inch cubes.

3. Place beef in a plastic bag with the flour mix; shake to coat the meat.

4. Set the Instant Pot to SAUTÉ and add olive oil.

5. Add the beef mixture, plus onion, shallots, and garlic. Sauté until the beef is lightly browned, or about 5 minutes.

6. Add broth, wine, vinegar, and dates. Stir to mix well.

7. Press CANCEL, close the lid, and cook at high pressure for 40 minutes.

8. When the cooking is complete, use a natural pressure release.

9. Serve beef over steamed vegetables or mashed potatoes.

Nutritional Information (Per Serving)

Calories: 672
Fat: 26.2 g
Sat Fat: 7.9 g
Carbohydrates: 26.2 g
Fiber: 2.9 g
Sugar: 16 g
Protein: 77.3 g
Sodium: 541 mg

Tasty Fish Stew

Makes 4 servings

Ingredients:
4 tablespoons olive oil, divided
1 medium onion, sliced
4 garlic cloves, minced
½ cup dry white wine
1 cup clam juice
2½ cup water
½ pound red potatoes, diced
1½ cups tomatoes, diced
Salt and pepper to taste
1½ pounds white fish (halibut, cod, sea bass, or tilapia), cut into 2" pieces
2 tablespoons fresh lemon juice
2 tablespoons fresh dill, chopped

Directions:
1. Set the Instant Pot to SAUTÉ and add 2 tablespoons olive oil.
2. Add onion and cook for about 3 minutes.
3. Add garlic and cook for about half a minute.

4. Add white wine to deglaze. Stir to keep any crisped pieces from sticking to the bottom. Keep stirring until the wine has evaporated.

5. Add clam juice, water, potatoes, tomatoes, salt, and pepper.

6. Press CANCEL, close the lid, and cook at high pressure for 5 minutes.

7. When the cooking is complete, do a quick pressure release.

8. Set the Instant Pot to SAUTÉ and allow the stew to simmer. Add the pieces of fish and continue to simmer for 5 minutes. Do not overcook the fish; it should flake easily but not be tough.

9. Press CANCEL, add lemon juice, fresh dill, and 2 tablespoons olive oil. Combine and serve.

Nutritional Information (Per Serving)
Calories: 457
Fat: 16.3 g
Sat Fat: 2.4 g
Carbohydrates: 30.7 g
Fiber: 5.1 g
Sugar: 10.7 g
Protein: 43.3 g

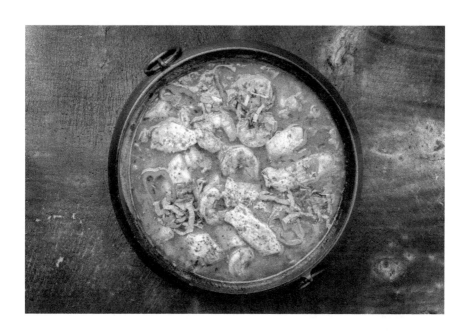

Coconut Curry Tilapia

Makes 4 servings

Ingredients:

1 tablespoon olive oil

½ teaspoon mustard seeds

½ inch slice of ginger, minced

3 cloves garlic, minced

8 mint leaves

2 teaspoons coriander

1 teaspoon cumin

1 teaspoon garam masala

½ teaspoon turmeric

1 teaspoon salt

½ medium onion, sliced

1 green pepper, sliced

1 red pepper, sliced

12 ounces coconut milk

1 pound tilapia, sliced into 2" pieces

3 sprigs cilantro

Directions:

1. Set the Instant Pot to SAUTÉ, and add olive oil and mustard seeds.

2. When you hear the seeds crackle, add ginger and garlic. Let sauté for 30 seconds.

3. Add onion and peppers, sauté for 30 seconds.

4. All mint leaves, coriander, cumin, garam masala, turmeric, and salt. Stir to mix. Cook for 30 seconds.

5. Add coconut milk and mix well. Bring the mixture to a simmer.

6. Add tilapia and cilantro. Stir well to make sure the fish is fully bathed in the curry mixture.

7. Press CANCEL, close the lid, and cook at high pressure for 3 minutes.

8. When the cooking is complete, do a quick pressure release.

Nutritional Information (Per Serving)
Calories: 348
Fat: 25.2 g
Sat Fat: 19 g
Carbohydrates: 10.8 g
Fiber: 3.5 g
Sugar: 5.5 g
Protein: 24.1 g
Sodium: 639 mg

Mediterranean Calamari

Makes 6 servings

Ingredients:

2 pounds calamari, chopped

2 tablespoons olive oil

1 red onion, sliced

3 cloves of garlic, chopped

1 cup red wine

3 stalks of celery, chopped

1 can (28 ounces) crushed tomatoes

3 sprigs fresh rosemary

½ cup Italian parsley, chopped

Salt and pepper to taste

Directions:

1. Toss the calamari pieces in olive oil and salt and pepper.

2. To the Instant Pot, add the wine, tomatoes with their juices, celery, rosemary, garlic, and red onion.

3. Place the calamari in a steamer basket and lower it to the liquid. Cook at high pressure for 4 minutes.

4. When the cooking is complete, use a natural pressure release.

5. Remove the fish and sprinkle with fresh parsley.

Nutritional Information (Per Serving)

Calories: 278

Fat: 6.9 g

Sat Fat: 1.2 g

Carbohydrates: 19.2 g

Fiber: 5 g

Sugar: 8.7 g

Protein: 27.3 g

Orange Salmon

Makes 4 servings

Ingredients:

1½ pounds salmon fillets

1 cup water

Salt and pepper to taste

4 teaspoons olive oil

1 medium onion, chopped

5 tablespoons parsley, chopped

2 teaspoons orange rind

Orange slices

Directions:

1. Insert a trivet in the Instant Pot and add the water.

2. Season the salmon fillets with salt, pepper, and olive oil, and arrange them on the trivet.

3. Place onion, parsley, and orange rinds on top of the salmon.

4. Close the lid, choose MANUAL, and cook at low pressure for 5 minutes.

5. When the cooking is complete, do a quick pressure release.

6. Garnish with orange slices and serve.

Nutritional Information (Per Serving)

Calories: 279

Fat: 15.2 g

Sat Fat: 2.2 g

Carbohydrates: 3.1 g

Fiber: 0.9 g

Sugar: 1.2 g

Protein: 33.4 g

Instant Pot Hummus

Makes 4 servings

Ingredients:

¾ cup dried chickpeas, rinsed

3 cups water

1 teaspoon salt

2 tablespoons olive oil

1 tablespoon lemon juice

1 garlic clove, minced

Pepper and parsley to taste

Directions:

1. Add chickpeas, salt, and water to the Instant Pot.

2. Close the lid and cook at high pressure for 45 minutes.

3. When the cooking is complete, do a natural pressure release for 10 minutes. Quick release the remaining pressure.

4. Using a colander, drain liquid from chickpeas, saving the cooking liquid for later use.

5. Add olive oil, lemon juice, garlic and ¼ cup of the cooking liquid to a food processor. Add the chickpeas and blend until creamy, adding more liquid as needed. Season to taste.

6. Serve with parsley.

Nutritional Information (Per Serving)
Calories: 199
Fat: 9.3 g
Sat Fat: 1.3 g
Carbohydrates: 23.1 g
Fiber: 6.6 g
Sugar: 4.1 g
Protein: 7.3 g
Sodium: 597 mg

Wine Poached Figs on Yogurt Crème

Makes 4 servings

Ingredients:

4 large sized figs

1 cup red wine

¼ cup honey

½ cup assorted nuts (chopped cashews, almonds, and pistachios)

4 cups plain yogurt

Directions:

1. Pour the yogurt into a mesh strainer and place it in the fridge to drain for about 6 hours. Do not wait for too long or the yogurt might get too crumbly.

2. Wash the figs and pat them dry. Place them in the Instant Pot. Add the wine and sugar and cover the lid of the pot.

3. Cook at high pressure for 6–7 minutes.

4. When the cooking is complete, use a natural pressure release.

5. On serving plates, add the yogurt crème, and poached figs. Garnish with wine syrup and chopped nuts on top.

Nutritional Information (Per Serving)
Calories: 358
Fat: 5.1 g
Sat Fat: 2.6 g
Carbohydrates: 49.3 g
Fiber: 2.4 g
Sugar: 45.5 g
Protein: 15.3 g
Sodium: 176 mg

Final Thoughts

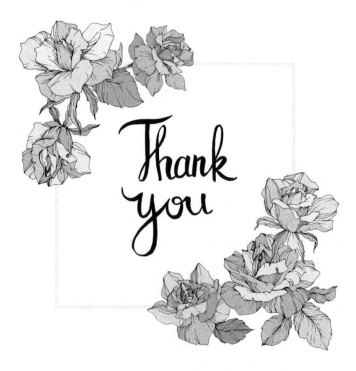

Finally, I want to thank you for reading my book. If you enjoyed the book, please take the time to share your thoughts and post a review on the book retailer's website. It would be greatly appreciated!

Best wishes,

Melinda Nelson

Lightning Source UK Ltd.
Milton Keynes UK
UKHW020033060620
364498UK00002B/326